THOUGHT CATALOG BOOKS

How To Sext

How To Sext

A Guide For Driving Your Man Crazy

THOUGHT CATALOG

THOUGHT CATALOG BOOKS

Brooklyn, NY

THOUGHT CATALOG BOOKS

Copyright © 2016 by The Thought & Expression Co.

All rights reserved. Published by Thought Catalog Books, a division of The Thought & Expression Co., Williamsburg, Brooklyn. Founded in 2010, Thought Catalog is a website and imprint dedicated to your ideas and stories. We publish fiction and non-fiction from emerging and established writers across all genres. For general information and submissions: manuscripts@thoughtcatalog.com.

First edition, 2016

ISBN 978-1530955770

10 9 8 7 6 5 4 3 2 1

Cover design by © Daniella Urdinlaiz

Contents

1

5 Steamy Reasons You Should Most Definitely Be Sexting

Samantha Podias

Living in a time where people are constantly on their phones can have its downsides, but this is definitely not one of them. Here are a few reasons why everyone should be hopping on the sexting train.

1. It's great foreplay.

When you're involved in any kind of sexual relationship with someone, foreplay is important because it's a starting point to get both you and your partner excited and ready for the next sexual act (whatever that may be). Sexting is an easy way (especially if you're in a long-distance relationship, or going long periods of time without physically seeing your partner) to get that arousal and excitement started with just the click of your "send" button. The anticipation of writing out and reading what you and your partner want to/will do to one another once you're together is such a turn on that by the time you're actually in the same room, you'll literally be ripping each other's clothes off.

2. It fosters communication about your desires.

In my own experience and in the experiences of my friends, I've found that often times what can make sex bad is a lack of communication or not feeling comfortable enough to tell your partner what you want (or don't want) during sex. Sexting is a perfect opportunity to be vocal and honest about your sexual desires, without the pressure of being face-to-face with your partner (or mid-sex) when you do it. Sexting beforehand will ensure that you and your partner know exactly what the other one wants sexually, so that once you're physically together, you won't waste any time worrying that what you're doing isn't pleasurable for both of you.

3. It's easy.

Although a lot of people will argue that this age of technology we're in is making us constantly stuck in our phones and disconnected from one another, it also makes communicating with one another extremely easy. Especially for those who are in long-distance relationships, sexting makes maintaining the sexual connection with your partner that much easier. Any time you have a spare moment, (when you're walking to class, on your lunch break, laying in your bed, etc.) you can literally send a sext to your partner in under a minute. With texting being as prevalent in our society as it is, we might as well take advantage of it and have ourselves some quick and easy dirty talk!

4. It's safer than actual sex.

Whenever you have sex (any kind of sex), it comes with unavoidable risks such as sexually transmitted diseases or pregnancy. When you sext, you can get down and dirty without worrying that either of these might be potential consequences. Similar to phone and Skype sex, sexting is so great because you can have an orgasm (or five) without even the slightest concern that you might contract an STD or become pregnant, which are big parts of what can make sex so complicated. Seems like a no-brainer to me!

5. It's just plain FUN!

Unless you are someone who legitimately doesn't enjoy dirty talk, there is no way that sexting will bring you anything but pure pleasure and enjoyment. The rush of having a filthy convo with your partner while sitting in your stat lecture is so exciting and can make just another dull Monday, extremely exhilarating. Some of the best sexts I've ever sent and received were while I was sitting in a boring class or taking a study break in the library. Sexts are a safe and easy way to get pleasure even while doing your most mundane activities, so go ahead and hit send!

2

10 Little Things That Make Your Man Ache For You (Even When You're Not Around)

Jillian Paulson

Men are like the easiest, simplest creatures in the world. They pretty much have three moods: horny, sleepy and hungry. You can appeal to all of these at the same time and keep his mind (and his boner) on your beautiful mind, face and body until he gets home and gives it to you.

1. Never forget the power of a strategic sext.

When my dude leaves me to go to work, I like to snap a photo of my undressed self still in bed and text it to him. I've successfully lured him back into my arms a few times with this method. Other good times to send something sexy? The 3 PM slump never fails.

2. A picture says 1,000 words.

Cue up "I Want a Little Sugar in my Bowl" and go to selfie-town. A particularly effective shot for certain men is just the top of your lacy panties, and another I've found gets great feedback is the underside of my boobs in a cropped sweater. Play around with angles and always send them his way for "critiques." No dude I know would be opposed to playing a little game of photography critic.

3. Take him online shopping with you.

I've been shopping for sexy Vegas dresses for an upcoming girlfriends trip, and I like to take my dude along by running a few options past him. Then I know he's thinking about me in that tight, white bodycon dress with the super-low neckline, which makes him think about my boobs in that dress, which makes him think of taking it off me, which makes him think of sex, which makes him think about cumming all over my tits. God, men are easy.

4. Keep him going on a few social media channels.

You have so many ways to contact him! To do it without being creepy, be strategic. Do you usually GChat during the day? Be a little naughty and send him a dirty message in the middle of your normal chatting. Send him an Instagram DM of your favorite lingerie or a handwritten note that says something sexy, even if it's just like "I can't wait to see you tonight" with a little winking drawing.

5. Be forthright.

I've never known a dude who didn't like it when I told him via text that I'd been thinking about choking on his cock all day. Don't beat around the (LOL) bush. Say what you're thinking about in as much dirty detail as you want. Another winner? "I can't stop thinking about how you bent me over and made me scream last night."

6. Send a screenshot.

A friend of mine sends her dude screenshots of the porn she's watching which is usually hot chicks playing with themselves. It's like a naughty little look into what turns her on, which of course turns him on.

7. Steal one of his white T-shirts and then wear it at least once a week in a new, sexy manner.

Like, wet in the shower. Or without pants. Send him photos of his shirt and all the adventures you two have together when he's not around.

8. Let him watch you get dressed for work in the morning.

He'll think about you putting on your clothes all day, and then he'll think about taking them off that evening. Bonus points if you choose a sexy black dress or pencil skirt.

9. Using your vibrator? Make a video.

Men love visual stimulation so they love any video you send. I promise. Even if it's you blowing a kiss. If you're really talented, bring the phone into the shower with you and send him a video of you soaping up.

10. If you wanna get romantic – and you should!

Dudes love romance! – send him a little love letter, or a love email. A sweet "I'm thinking about you" reminder keeps you in his brain and his heart (awwww!) all day.

3

15 Tips For Taking Killer Nudes

Jillian Paulson

Wait a minute! Who is leaking MY nude photos? If those celeb nude photos, supposedly "deleted" but leaked via a flaw in the iCloud, got released, then where the hell are mine?

Mine are super good! I don't have someone handy to TAKE them because duh, I'm single, but I do a pretty good job with the TimerCam app and the selfie flip on my phone. I mean, Jennifer Lawrence's are pretty sexy, and Kate Upton's boobs look exactly as awesome as I thought they would, but I think my naked selfies are pretty legit. They're just floating around in cyberspace in that "cloud" that literally no one understands, I guess. Well, if they end up in your hands, have fun!

You wanna take the perfect nudies to send to whoever via text message? Have I got some tips for you.

1. Don't go fully naked. I mean, do you really want to send a full-frontal totally-naked shot to someone? No, you don't. Start with a nipple, or even the suggestion of boobs with a bare shoulder or a sheer tee.

2. Stay within your comfort zone. No person is worth you feeling ashamed or nervous. If you don't feel comfortable sending them photos, do not do it.

3. Know your angles. Do you look best from the left side? Then always aim to show that off. Also, an angled body tends to look slimmer and more flattering.

4. Butt selfies are really hard. I'm still trying to master this, but I have found they look best when shot kneeling, with the camera flipped "selfie style" and held low, but angled. Your butt looks bigger that way, and any cellulite is hidden by the reverse camera. Twisting around is tough, though. Hold the pose, America's Next Top Model!

5. One of my go-to pics is just the top of whatever underwear I'm wearing that day. For some reason, just the pic of my navel ring and some lace-topped underwear sends dudes into a frenzy.

6. Another good one is the bath photo. Droplets of water, or suds, on your skin is always sexy.

7. Accentuate your best assets. Mine are my boobs. I generally always focus on boobs.

8. KEEP YOUR SOCKS OUT OF THE PHOTO.

9. Hard nipples = always better.

10. Lighting is key. You don't want FULL light, but if it's too dark, what's the point? And always, always, refrain from using the flash.

11. If you're taking a mirror photo, clean the mirror off, please.

12. Don't show your face unless you really trust the person. I'm just saying that sometimes shit happens and things get sent around. Then again, don't send nudes to someone you don't trust, either. Unless you don't care about it, and then by all means, send away.

13. Be a tease. The top of a stocking, a bare leg or just the hint of nipples through a T-shirt can be way sexier than a totally naked pic.

14. Send 'em to your girlfriends for critiques. I do this. Getting sexy pics from my girls is fun, and it's a good way to build up confidence.

15. Make YOURSELF feel sexy. Wear what makes YOU feel good, and it'll show through in your pictures. And if all else fails, black lace is a good place to start.

4

100 Things You Should Sext Your Man If You Want Him To Cum In His Pants Immediately

Adrienne West

1. Why aren't you cumming down my throat right now?

2. Even when you're not here you give me the best orgasms.

3. I'm naked in bed waiting for you.

4. I want your cum dripping out of me.

5. Just so you know, you can cum anywhere, anytime.

6. You make me so wet.

7. Can you please cum on my tits next time?

8. I miss your cock.

9. I'm stressed. I need you to fuck me until I can't remember my name.

10. I've never been this wet before.

11. My pussy misses you.

12. I want to do something with you sexually you've never done before.

13. I just thought about you and I swear I got wet immediately.

14. My nipples get hard when you text me.

15. It's been so long since I've sucked on your balls.

16. I don't know why, but all I could think about in my work meeting was kneeling in front of you and getting you off.

17. I can't wait to get home so I can sit on your face.

18. I'm sore in the best way from last night.

19. If I come to your office for lunch, which way do you want to fuck me on your desk first?

20. All I can think about is how you taste.

21. I just came so hard thinking about the way you pull my hair when you fuck me.

22. I'm not wearing panties today.

23. I'm ruining the panties I wore today thinking about you.

24. I just got a wax, wanna see?

25. I get to suck you dry before we go out tonight.

26. I miss hearing you cum.

27. Pretty sure my neighbors can hear when I think about you.

28. If you say one more thing I'm going to have to finish myself right here right now.

29. Is it wrong that just seeing those blue dots next to your name gets me wet?

30. Your cock is literally perfect.

31. Just so you know, you can have me any way, any time.

32. I'm at work and all I can think about is your cock.

33. How many times do you think I can make you cum tonight?

34. I couldn't decide which panties you'd like best, so I decided not to wear any.

35. Can I give you head while you play video games later?

36. You have no idea how bad I want you to fuck me right now.

37. As soon as you walk in the door tonight I'm getting on my knees.

38. I was looking at my tits in the mirror and thinking about how much better they'd look with your cum on them.

39. Why aren't you fucking me right now?

40. You make me think the nastiest thoughts.

41. I'm really craving your cum right now.

42. You made me make such a mess in my bed.

43. You made me cum so hard last time I swear I was going to pass out.

44. How long am I supposed to wait until I tell you how much I want your cock again?

45. You fuck me so good.

46. I just made myself cum thinking about you, but I'm down for round 2 if you feel like coming over.

47. Your cock drives me crazy.

48. I think it would be really hot if I could tie you up and tease you for hours before I make you cum.

49. I keep thinking about the way your cum tastes. I need to taste it again.

50. I think I'm in love with your cock.

51. I would suck your dick every morning if I could.

52. I wanna see your handprint on this ass.

53. You're not leaving your bed this weekend.

54. I could never get tired of fucking you.

55. Ever since I met you I can't stop touching myself whenever I'm in bed.

56. I wish you knew all the bad things I want to do to you tonight.

57. I ordered us a new toy.

58. I never knew I was so perverted until I met you and you made me think of all the ways I want you to make me cum.

59. Can you be showered and in sweats by 8? I have a list of naughty things I want to do to you tonight.

60. Cum over and don't say anything, I want to blow you for at least a half hour before I make you cum harder than you ever have before.

61. No one makes my panties wet like you.

62. Pull my hair tonight.

63. When is a good time to tell you how bad I want you to fuck me from behind right now?

64. Just so you know I'm going to make you cum at least twice when you get home tonight.

65. I just read that semen is supposed to be good for your skin. Can we test it out later?

66. I have expensive whiskey and I want you.

67. I love how sexy you look when you're making me cum.

68. I was just thinking about how hard you made me cum last time. When can I see you?

69. I can't decide if I want you to cum in my mouth or in my pussy more.

70. Fresh from church and ready 2 sin.

71. Can we go skinny dipping?

72. Here's a picture of my boobs just because.

73. Here's a picture of the panties I was wearing before I got them too wet thinking about you.

74. I can't stop thinking about what you feel like when you're inside me.

75. Tonight: fuck me like you hate me.

76. Tonight: make me cum while your cock is in my mouth.

77. Don't talk tonight, just lay back and let me do all the work.

78. The only words I'm going to say tonight are 'yes sir.'

79. Cum over.

80. Your hands and your dick can do no wrong.

81. I'm not usually this horny. But here I am sending you sexts in the middle of the afternoon because you've turned me into such a slut.

82. I'd give up Netflix forever just to feel your fingers on my clit right now.

83. I'm dripping wet for you.

84. I could explain how horny you make me, but I'd rather you stick your fingers inside me and feel for yourself.

85. I want my tongue over every inch of your cock and balls.

86. I want to sit on your face until I can't cum anymore.

87. You know what happens when you first get inside me? That's all I've thought about at work today.

88. I need a good fucking.

89. I want to cum for you so badly.

90. I wish I was waking you up with a BJ right now.

91. Spank me later?

92. Be naked when I get home.

93. You. Me. No clothes. All weekend.

94. You've turned me into such a dirty little slut.

95. I need your tongue on my clit immediately.

96. I get turned on just thinking about your cum on me.

97. Tonight I'm going to tease you until you fucking beg to cum.

98. Last night I got myself off thinking about how I want to choke on your cock tonight.

99. The only thing that's getting me through this day is the thought of your tongue on my clit.

100. You made me work all day in wet panties.

5

'H' Is For Hard: A Sexting Alphabet

Jillian Paulson

Last night I was awakened with a story idea, and the little bird of inspiration wouldn't be satisfied until I woke my ass up and wrote it down on my phone to revisit in the morning. What was that oh-so-important idea; the one that woke me from my slumber just so I could give it its due?

"The A-Z of sexting."

Yep, that's right. "Jillian, write about sexting again!" chirped the inspiration bird. "You know all about it! You're basically an encyclopedia of dick pics and easy ways to get a dude all turned on and shit! Why not share your wisdom with others?"

Not a bad idea, honestly. Open up your notebooks, students, and let's get to work.

A is for Angles.

If you're sending a sexy photo to someone, it's good to know your best angles. For girls, lying on your stomach and taking a photo of your ass in cute underwear always works. For dudes, figure out which poses make your junk look its most appetizing.

B is for Booty Call, which is what sexting often leads to.

Sometimes, though, sexting can replace the act of the booty call. You can get off "with" someone without having to have another person in your space.

C is for Critique my dick pic, the ultimate resource for taking the best dick shot you possibly can.

Run by @moscaddie, it's a crucial reference manual for literally any dude. She critiques dicks with love and a trained eye.

D is for Dirty.

Tell that dude you want him to drag his cum across your face. Why not?

E is for Enthusiasm.

No one likes having sex with a dead fish! And no one likes sexting with one, either. Don't be half-assed about it. E is also for Emoji; it's not nice to respond to nudes or sexy texts with only an emoji.

F is for Fun.

Because sexting is fun. It's pretty much the most fun you can have on your phone besides playing the Kim Kardashian Hollywood game. It's like foreplay that you can do (basically) alone, so it's perfect for introverts!

G is for Garters.

A flash of stockings and garters via photo or video is like an instant boner for most dudes. It's OK if you, like me, only wear them for about 5 minutes before yanking them off.

H is for Hard.

Dicks get hard, obviously, and talking about how hard you are/how hard a dude was is an easy, never-fail sext. But also, sexting can be kind of hard – don't resort to clichés like "I'm going to fuck the shit out of you." Don't get stuck in Hackneyed (HA HA) descriptions and similes.

I is for Initiate.

Who starts the sexting? How do you even start? Maybe you recently had really good sex with this person and you want to repeat it. Text them that you can't stop thinking about when they _____. If you look really good that day, send a little teaser photo and get the ball rolling by hinting at what's underneath.

J is for Jerkin' It

AKA what you do with your favorite sexts and/or videos after the fact when you need extra masturbatory material. Plus, asking "Are you touching yourself?" is always hot.

K is for Kinky.

One of my dude friends said the best sext he ever got from a girl included her requesting that he "tie me up and tell me what a dumb slut I am." Even if you don't actually carry this out, it's still fun to fantasize about.

L is for Lame Sexting.

Dudes, going "what would u do to me if I was there lol" is not sexy. It's boring, it's half-assed and it puts all the focus on you. Don't be a lazy ass.

M is for Mistakes.

Be sure you're sexting the right person and not your room-mate, coworker or a family member. It can happen!

N is for Natural Light.

It's always best. Don't send me a pic of your dick in a dark room like you're a troll or a mushroom. Use light to your advantage.

O is for One-Handed Typing.

Which is what you're doing if your sext session is working.

P is for Privacy.

Don't put your face in your nudies if you're worried about the other party sharing them.

Q is for Questions.

A little sexy Q & A is fun and informative. You can figure out what your partner likes simply by playing a game of 20 Questions.

R is for Reciprocate.

Studies show that women are more likely to send sexy texts than men. Ladies, it's not fair that dudes get to receive all the fun photos and texts you're sending; they need to give it right back. Sexting is a two-person game.

?S is for Spell Check.

Get it right, get it tight. (That sort of applies, right?)

T is for Tits.

They never fail. You've got a great pair, so show them off. A few classic poses include:
• Arm over bare chest
• Bra pulled down so just a little bit of nipple shows
• Bra half-on, half-off
• Tan lines. (This is my go-to.)

U is for Unique.

Sext like you talk. Don't get too flowery, because no one wants a Danielle Steel novel in their text messages. Be yourself!

V is for Videos.

Never underestimate the power of a sexy video. Another dude friend once got a video of a girl doing yoga poses naked and he "jacked it a million times to that one."

W is for "Wet."

Why is wet such a sexy word? Saying how wet you are/how wet you want to make your partner is simple and forthright. Also, sending photos when you're actually wet, like emerging from the shower or lying in the bath, is never a bad call.

X is for X-rated.

What else would it stand for? It's just texting, so get as dirty as you want. Use words you might not say out loud. Go crazy.

Y is for You're Hot!

Don't be shy. The person on the receiving end of your sexts thinks you're hot as balls, so embrace it!

Z is for ... jiZZ? (OK, I tried.)

6

15 People Share The Cringeworthy Details Of Their Most Mortifying Sexting Fail

Becca Martin

1. "I was Snapping my girlfriend a picture with my shirt off that said "hehe" but I ended up sending it to her little sister. My girlfriend's sister asked her about it, I would rather buy a one way ticket to Europe and never come back instead of seeing her again."

– Jacob, 21

2. "When I was drunk I was sending naked Snapchats to my boyfriend but accidentally sent them to my family's foreign exchange student. I called my younger sister, who was at my parent's house with him, and made her go to his room while he was sleeping and open them all so he'd never see them."

– Kylie, 20

3. "My girlfriend didn't answer her phone when I called her, but I was away on business so I was horny and missed her.

Since she didn't answer her phone so I left her a voicemail. She listened to it through her car Bluetooth with her mom in the car. I don't know who it was more awkward for."

– Blake, 26

4. "I took naked posed pictures to send to this guy I was talking to, but forgot my phone automatically syncs when it's hooked up to my computer. So the pictures were now on my laptop, which my dad later saw. It was the most awkward encounter in my life. I would rather do just about anything than have anything like that ever happen again in my life."

– Michelle, 19

5. "In 9th grade I was texting this girl with a foot fetish and she sent me nudes for a couple pictures of my ankles."

– Tony, 23

6. "I accidentally put a nude on my Snap story instead of sending it to the person it would as intended for. Like 10 people saw it before anyone let me know it was up. Luckily no family members saw it, but it was so embarrassing."

– Sarah, 22

7. "Set a Snapchat of me fingering myself as my story for about 12 minutes. Whoops!"

– Kim, 24

8. "One time I was talking to this guy, and we were Snapchatting so I decided to sent him a nude. The one time I decided to, I actually accidentally sent the naked Snapchat to my cousin. My cousin's name was right above this guy in my Snapchat contacts. I was naked from head to toe and it was so obvious who it was. The worst part it, my cousin answered when he was drunk and told me I was 'sexy af' AWKWARD."

– Vanessa, 21

9. "Accidentally sent a super dirty text to my high school basketball coach…"

– Keri, 23

10. "One time in middle school, I went to go take a picture (on my Blackberry) for a guy. I didn't have a mirror in my bedroom so I went into the bathroom and climbed up on the side of the bathtub to take a picture. I took one and the sound was on and my mom asked me what I was doing and I told her I had a big poop and had to show my friend."

– Liz, 25

11. "In high school I used to take pictures of my iPod touch and have to send them to my email to email to my phone because I didn't have a front camera. One day my mom went through my iPod and saw all my naked pictures and called me out on it. She asked me so many questions and all I could do was laugh because it was so awkward."

– Melissa, 22

12. "My mom found my phone and read my sexts. She told me it was worse than *50 Shades of Grey* and my little sister started crying."

– Brooke, 21

13. "My dad meant to send a dirty text to my mom about what they were going to do after work, but sent it to me instead. I'm a dude and it was still weird...but hey good for him that he's still getting it."

– Billy, 24

14. "I got really fucked up and I wanted to make my ex-boyfriend jealous so I told his friend to write his name on my tits, and he did. But he also took a picture of it and made it his Twitter header."

– Marley, 21

15. "I was blacked out and I thought it would be funny to take a Snapchat video of me doing this girl from behind, but instead of sending it to my friend I put in on my story. She had no idea and I didn't realize it until the morning. A bunch of people texted me that night, but I passed out after the sex."

– Chris, 25

7

How To Live Your Best Life And Spend Thanksgiving Secretly Sexting At Your Family Party

Adrienne West

The whole point of sexting is that it's supposed to be fun and scandalous. It's the anticipation of something you want and can't have. Personally, my favorite time to sext is in the morning when I wake up because my boyfriend is already at his office and I know he's going to see the Snapchat notification and be dying to find a time and place to watch it. And *then* he'll actually see it and feel things he won't be able to act on for hours. By the time we see each other we're both keyed up and dying to touch one another. Actually, it's gotten us into the weird (but really fun) routine of trading oral as soon as we see each other and then talking about our days, making dinner, doing the usual end of day things afterwards.

If you've been together a long time, chances are you are spending Thanksgiving with them. If that's the case, here's a guide for having discreet sex at your parent's house.

However if you're single or seeing someone new, don't waste the opportunity to turn a mundane family event into something that pushes you both to the edge of anticipation and unable to wait to see each other again.

Start when he has downtime.

Sexting is all about the build-up. You need to set the tone for the day before he's in the thick of it with his family. If you know his dinner starts at 6, for instance, send your first sext at 5. Make sure he goes into his day with you on his mind. Send him a snap of you dressing for your dinner, or just tell him "I don't know why because there's nothing sexy about this holiday, but all I can think about this morning is how bad I wanna get you off."

Don't rely on him responding to feel good about yourself.

That said, family days can get crazy or they can have a ton of downtime with your phone and you don't always know how it's going to be in advance. If he isn't responding right away, don't get your feelings hurt and let it ruin your day. Maybe he's out tossing a football in the yard with his little cousins. Maybe his mom is making him help with the turkey. You don't know what's going on on the other end of the line so focus on the pleasure *you* get from teasing him and doing something a little naughty at whatever family house you're at.

If he is responding, make sure your sound is off when you watch his snaps.

Write the perfect text.

The perfect text really depends on the person receiving it. What kind of relationship do you have? Have you already slept together? Are you trying to tease them subtly or explicitly?

I asked some of my guy friends to see what the best text sexts they've ever received were:

"I want you inside me"

"I'm sorry if this is too much, but I get wet any time I think about you."

"Can you do that thing you did to me again? I swear I couldn't remember my name for like 30 minutes"

"All I can think about right now is you inside me"

"I swear to god I had the sexiest dream of my life about you last night and if you don't act it out with me in the next 24 hours I'm going to combust."

"I'm really worked up today, can I stop by on my break and give you a BJ?"

"I can't believe you made me work the last 3 hours of my day with wet panties"

"I want you to blindfold me and then cum wherever you want to"

"Why is the only thing I can think about today the way your face looks when your dick is in my mouth?"

Don't underestimate the power of video.

Sending stills in Snapchat is the easiest thing to do. You can find a great angle, take the picture and be done with it. Video can be awkward because you have less control over how the finished product looks, plus, what are you supposed to do? You're smiling for a few minutes or just moving the camera over a body part or two. It doesn't feel natural.

BUT videos are SO much better! It makes you feel like you are right there with the person. It's much more enticing and hot. And when you see a video of someone, you never think it's weird or awkward the way you feel making it.

Bathrooms (with locks) are your friend.

You can spend most of the day teasing through text or sending PG Snapchat stills with x-rated text overlays. But every once in awhile you need to break it up. Sneak off to the bathroom and capture the goods on camera. The fact that you're sneaking off to send him these pics when you're supposed to be a good girl and helping out with whatever family stuff will drive him crazy.

8

Everything You've Ever Wanted To Know About Sexting And Sending Dick Pics (But Were Afraid To Ask)

Jillian Paulson

So you've been texting with a new dude and said texts have now progressed past flirtatious and are just flat-out sexts. Awesome. But are you a little clueless as to how to interpret said sexts? What does that dude actually mean when he's saying all those things?

Luckily I am the Queen of Sexting and I can interpret these confusing messages for you. Sit down, students, and learn. Perhaps we should call this Sexting 101?

Part One: Sexual Emojis

The "water droplets" Emoji: Either means squirting or jizz
Eggplant emoji: Boners

Peach (fruit) emoji: Butt

Tongue: Clearly this means oral sex (This one squicks me out HARDCORE)

Tongue + droplets: Female oral sex

Blushing face: You're turning me on AND freaking me out

Hearts-in-eyes face: I am loving everything you're saying

Part Two: What Does He Actually Mean?

"I'm so hard right now."

Translation: I'm probably a little bit hard but I'm at work/ school/using public transportation, so I'm trying not to get actually hard because that's embarrassing.

"I bet you look hot right now."

Translation: Send me a picture of your boobs.

"Your tits are so nice."

Translation: Send me more pictures of your boobs.

"I'm drunk."

Translation: Let's bone. I'm using this as an excuse to say things to you that I wouldn't say sober.

"I'm gonna fuck you so hard."

Translation: I'm in my pajamas eating nachos, not actively thinking about fucking you.

"What do you wanna do to me right now?"

Translation: You do all the work here. I'm lazy and want to get off without a whole lot of work fantasizing on my own.

Part Three: Dick Pic Pet Peeves

I don't actually care what your dick looks like. I only like what it can DO to me. That said, if you really feel inclined to show me what it looks like …

DON'T

1. Include your socks. (This might be a personal pet peeve.)
2. EVER send a flaccid one.
3. Use the TV remote as a measurement device.
4. Send a picture using your dirty bathroom mirror.
5. Make it shiny. Ew.
6. Use MONEY to measure it. I do not want to see $2 in quarters on your fucking dick. MONEY IS DIRTY. I am not impressed by its length; I'm grossed out thinking of all the hands that touched that money. That shit is NOT going in my mouth without a proper sanitation.
7. Send them out of the blue. If I haven't seen it in person, I don't want to see it on the phone.
8. Include your face. HELLO, I can send this to my friends. And I probably will if it's particularly a) impressive or b) hilarious.
9. No wedding rings, please.

DO

1. Reference the situation in some manner. We're texting and you get hard? Show me.

2. Keep a little bit of hair down there. A shaved dick area freaks me out.

3. Be tasteful. I don't mind a little bit of light stroking via video.

4. Consider lighting. Natural light is best.

5. Find your angles. Don't make it look tiny!

6. Consider the backdrop. I can SEE the lady razor in your shower and I know you don't have a girl roommate!

7. Ask before you send. Seriously. Be considerate. I know that you'd be happy getting 100,000 surprise pics of my vagina, but you won't be, so settle your ass down. Just don't blast a dick pic to me in the middle of the day when I'm in line at Starbucks. I will show the barista.

Part Four: Foolproof Sexting Ideas

• Boobs. Use the flip cam for the best angle. Plus, then you don't need to show your face. Always have hard nipples, because they photograph better.

• "Oh my god" is much sexier than any other phrase when you're strapped for anything creative to say.

• "And then what?" usually gets you a good story.

• Dudes are visual. Send them a video every once in awhile if you trust them. I like a good "soaping up the boobs," but I'm good at holding my phone in the bathtub. Don't try that if you're clumsy.

• Know that he will probably show SOMEONE. Therefore, don't send anything you're not comfortable with.

• Know you look hot? Take a picture. It'll make his day, even if it's just a picture of your shoes.

• I am not ashamed of using the "winky" face. It conveys flirting.

• Don't sext with anyone you don't trust. I have to say this a few times for your protection. If anything, SCREENSHOT THAT SHIT when he sends you a bad dick pic so you can use it one day if you need to. I mean … never mind.

<u>9</u>

10 Ways You And Your Partner Can Have A Healthier Sext Life

Sarah Packard

1. Make sure it's the right place and right time

The best thing about sexting is that you can literally do it any-time and anywhere, but therein lies the problem. You never quite know what's happening on the other side of that phone. Sure, a little teasing to spice up a dull work day can be exciting, but no one wants a dick pic popping up on their iPhone in the middle of a boardroom. And you might be feeling randy, but no one ever wants to send a perfectly crafted dirty text only to receive a response of "At temple with Grandma." Oy! That's why your safest sext is usually the late-night one. Make sure the other person is at home, alone, and most importantly in the mood.

2. Don't start something you can't finish

In this day and age it seems we always have to be doing a thou-sand things at once. While you may have sexted while watching TV, surfing the internet, or cleaning your house (gross), the only thing that truly matters is that you're willing to stick around for a bare minimum of 20 minutes. If you're about to run out the door to meet friends do NOT engage. If you're about to take an hour long shower do NOT get him going. And for the love of God please don't start and then fall asleep. There's nothing more humiliating than to be completely left hanging.

3. It's all about the innuendo

Just like in actual sex, you've often got to dip your toes in and get a little wet before jumping right in. That's when the Art of the innuendo comes into play. Think of it as the foreplay of sexting. And don't worry if you're not a master of the written word. In fact, it's best to keep it short and sweet. As you become more experienced, you soon realize you can make LITERALLY ANYTHING SEXUAL.

She texts, "OMG I just had my ass kicked at CrossFit!" You can respond, "But I thought you liked it a little rough..."

He asks, "How about this rain, huh?" You can say "Yeah...now I'm really soaking wet."

And you'll never go wrong texting your man a simple, "Working hard??" for a little midday pick-me-up.

It's simple as that! Now, if you genuinely lack all creativity and imagination you can always default with the classic winky face. Seriously, add it to anything. It's juvenile, but it works.

One last thing I must mention on this topic: For the love of GOD please nix the emojis from your sexting vocabulary. No self-respecting woman will ever be turned on by a spraying eggplant!

4. Be picky with your pics

They say a picture is worth a thousand words, but it can also be worth a thousand regrets. Of course, the seriousness of your relationship and the amount of trust you've built together are factors at play. If you're in a monogamous relationship, then I say Photoshop your privates all day if you want! But if your connection is on the newer side, it's always wise to use a bit more discretion. And if you haven't even met one another yet, then don't even THINK about it! It's no different than having something leaked to the internet; those pictures can last forever! And in the wrong hands they could really come back to haunt you.

5. On that note, guys... it's not really doing it for us

Look, I get it, men are visual creatures. But you must then remember that women are verbal ones. So guys, a pic of your little pecker isn't going to excite us nearly as much as you saying, "You looked so sexy and beautiful the other night…" And as much as you guys don't want to hear this— to us they really do all look the same. I'd say nine times out of ten it's actually more of a turn-off than a turn-on. What if we haven't even met Mr. Salami in person yet? Is that how you want first introductions to be? I say keep it in your pants and just tell us we're pretty.

6. Be a good conversationalist

A good sexting session is just like a good conversation: one person talks and the other listens.

Try to stay on message and don't interrupt. The same principles apply here. Often times the more verbose and imaginative one will lead the conversation. This is exactly what you want, because, as we all know, the worst kind of sexual experience is a vanilla one. If you happen to be on the receiving end of a verbose sexter, it's best to just sit back and enjoy the ride. Let them lead— it's what they want! The most important thing to remember is when you see that ellipse– DO NOT INTER-RUPT.

However, feel free to selectively interject throughout the spiel to help move things along and give your partner proper validation. You can stick with simple (but effective) responses such as "Oh YES," "Oh my God," or "I Love that." Or take it a step further with a rousing "What else do you want to do to me???" or a salacious "Baby that feels sooooo good." The possibilities are endless, and in the more passive role it's almost impossible to say the wrong thing.

7. Double check it before you sext it

It happens to us all: You're in the midst of a steamy sexting session. Emotionally charged and typing furiously while "multi-tasking" the absolute worst happens: your fingers slip and that Auto Correct devil rears its ugly, cock-blocking little head. Sometimes if it's a small enough blunder you can both let it slide. But other times all it takes is an "Mmm" to come out as "Mom" to really kill that mood.

"Oh baby, I want to duck you all night long" is sure to incite more giggles than it will 'gasms.

And trust me- no one's going to be turned on by your "big throbbing couch."

Also remember to double check that contact name so that you don't end up sexting your boss. Unless, of course, you're into that sort of thing ?

8. You always need a beginning, middle and an end

While some may argue the most important part of the modern day sext is the big finish, without a sufficient amount of build-up or at least some sort of story line, it's going to fall flat. I'll never forget the worst sexting experience of my life. I was getting ready for bed when a guy I'd been dating sent me an unsolicited picture of his aroused member with no textual explanation whatsoever. Then after five minutes of pregnant silence Casanova texted back "That was great- I needed that…."

I sat there dumbfounded. Was he SERIOUS?! That was IT??

To make matters worse he went on to ask, "So... did you enjoy that?"

All I could do was laugh. Enjoy what exactly?! I wasn't even aware I was taking part in anything! At that point I'd already put on pajamas and was watching True Detective. But since I was tired and didn't want him to feel badly, I texted back a winky face and then broke it off a week later.

9. Be sweet and delete

Unless you're a Snapchatting sexter, (which really is a different animal all together,) you should maybe think about deleting your naughtiest textual trysts. The scary thing is that nowadays anything you say over text actually CAN be held against you. I mean it's all right there... just scroll up. While there's absolutely nothing wrong with a little consensual dirty talk, it could potentially get you into a lot of trouble when it's out of context or in the wrong hands. If you happen to use the same device for both your personal and work phone you may want to do a little clean up. Or if you're now in a completely new relationship (especially with a confirmed snooper) you should probably get rid of those old messages ASAP. If you'd feel uncomfortable having your new partner or your entire IT department read it, then delete it.

10. When in doubt, just LIE YOU'RE ASS OFF

Not only do you not have to leave your house to successfully sext, you don't even have to brush your hair! It's all about fantasy…aka everyone is completely bs-ing each other. If you really are rocking out that sexy little matching baby doll set, then GOD BLESS YOU! But if you're a normal person and haven't showered all day and wearing some old, stained over-sized T shirt, then guess what?! He don't gots to know!!! This is when you lie, lie, lie, and then lie some more! That's the magic of sexting. You feel bad about being dishonest? Well believe you me– your partner's doing the same exact thing.

<u>10</u>

5 Simple Rules For Sexting

Kat George

1. Straight Girls Don't Like Dick Pics

Based on every straight girl I've ever spoken to, we, as a group, do not like dick pics. Dicks are not that pretty to begin with, and the from below angles of sext photos often make dicks look more like a monster attacking a city than an actual sexual organ. Straight dudes: you've been told.

2. Never, EVER Show Anyone Sexts You Got

Sexts are private. When someone agrees to give you their body, they agree to give YOU their body, not you and all your friends. It's a violation of privacy and trust to share sexts that someone entrusted to you, and only a really horrible person would do that to someone they care about. Showing off a sext is the fastest way to never get another sext again–and the fastest way to have the person that sext you cut you out of their life forever.

3. Make Sure You Look Hot (Just In Case)

It's all well and good to trust that your partner isn't showing off your sexts, but you never know what might happen in the case of an acrimonious break up. Showing off someone's sexts in revenge is the lowest of low, but if you wind up really hurting someone, you don't know what they might do to get back at you. Make sure you look damn fine in all your sext photos—just in case.

4. Check And Double Check Who You Are Sending To

Study the "to" field in your text. You don't want to be accidentally sending photos of your tits to your mom or boss.

5. Only Send To Someone You Trust

I send my boyfriend sexts because I trust him. I trust they're not going to end up in the public domain, I trust that he's not going to share them with his buddies, and I know that he's not going to mock me. There's a mutual respect involved in sexting—you want to know and trust the person you're sharing with, to avoid any negative consequences. Of course, some people engage in sexting very casually, and that's fine too, but always just be sure your expectations are commensurate with the intention on the other end.

11

5 Tips For Safely And Effectively Sexting With Snapchat

Matt Powers

Sexting is a dangerous game for both parties. For men, it's like confusing a pair of navy slacks for black ones; it just looks different with that lighting. For women it's like sitting on a tarped hill listening to Charlie Hunnam read *50 Shades of Grey*; you might get caught slippin'.

In light of the recent celebrity nude outrage, we're all scratching our heads wondering if the age of sexting is coming to an end, but the brave people at Snapchat continue to fight the good fight by deleting our pics, so here's how to make sure you're safe *and* effective:

1. Establish An Audience

You can't just Snap-sext willy-nilly. Like advertising, you have to establish a demand — unless it's your significant other, in which case there aren't really rules in regards to frequency and content. If you're single and on the conservative side, it might be three potentials, and if you're like me, you've relied on the best option: crowdsourcing.

To crowdsource, you simply send a Snapchat of yourself covered with a towel or something to all of your followers, with the caption, "The next one's nude ;)" After they open it, send another one and say, "Just kidding, but the next one really is ;)"

Note the amount of time people took to open your second Snap, the ones who opened it without hesitation are your fans.

2. Limit Your Snap's Time

One possible downside of Snapchat is that it can't stop the user from screenshotting your sext; that's why you need to play it safe by limiting it to a ONE second view time, because that's hardly long enough to pull off the two-hand *or* one-hand-claw screenshot. I also recommend imposing a strict zero-tolerance, 'one strike you're out' policy.

Once you and your fans establish a mutual trust, you can spoil them with a three second Snap.

3. Never Use Flash

Nothing makes you look more pale and corpse-like than flash, it's too reminiscent of those Polaroids used in abduction films. If your roommate sees a flash in the space below your door, it's just obvious and maybe not that classy. Fluorescent light isn't doing you any favors either, so your best bet is a soft, over-head, incandescent light-source. I mean, that's Indoor Photography 101.

4. Be Careful

The most unfortunate mistake, and one I've seen take place, is adding your sext to your Snapchat 'story.' Now all your friends and family can see your sext, but worse than that, your loyal fans who pride themselves on exclusivity will feel cheated.

5. Mix It Up

Absence makes the heart grow fonder, so drag out the suspense, send them one of your face to remind them who you are. Blow their minds; take a picture with Photo Booth that includes both of your hands, print it out and take a Snap-sext of that image so they'll wonder, "How the hell did they do that? Who took that picture?!" By the time your fans see it, it'll be too late for them to figure it out.

12

The Perks Of A Quick Sunday Sext

Jillian Paulson

You know, sometimes a good "Come over and fuck me fast before work" is the best thing imaginable.

Perhaps you've been batting sexy texts back and forth for a few days – pics of his morning wood, you finally learning how to take the perfect butt selfie. But your schedules just don't align right to get you both in the same (bed)room for more than half an hour.

I mean, I love a lengthy sex session as much as the next girl. I love when they spend time worshipping my entire body and giving me head as long as I like – hey, I can be greedy, but I always return the favor. It's super fun to have a few hours just to fuck around, from drawn-out foreplay to boning and then maybe doing it all again if dude can make it work.

But sometimes, as a Career Girl (LOL), you don't have time for that shit. You've got work to do, happy hours to attend, bottles of champagne to polish off at Sunday brunch. There's no room for a good deep-dicking in your busy schedule! And so you spend all day sending sneaky peeks of your cute outfit, the lingerie under it and the boobs under that lingerie, to that dude til he's so fired up he has no choice but to get in his car and drive to your Ivory Tower to give it to you.

I always thought it might be kinda fun to have a weekly-ish sex date with some dude I was sexually engaged to. You know: "Come over every Thursday at 9 PM until further notice." Wouldn't that be nice? It would be something to look forward to all week, for starters. "Oh, this week we're gonna do bondage shit. Last week we just played with my vibrator for like two hours." I'm a busy girl lately, so you gotta put it in my calendar if you wanna put it in me!

Generally on Sundays I prefer a dose of morning sex before we laze around all day, but since my current dude is decidedly NOT my boyfriend that ain't happening. So after I rolled home after mixing and matching various mixers with a full bottle of champagne at brunch with my bestie, I was just revved up enough to really want a little sex. And dude was down. "Are you alone? Should I come fuck u?" I might as well have answered, "Uh, duhhhh." I sometimes do.

So he shows up and I greet him at my door in my prettiest, fanciest and therefore most uncomfortable bra, which he swoons over and then rips off. And then it's like "Bam!" In my bedroom.

It's funny how you can pack all the necessary elements of a good sexing into a handful of minutes if you're dedicated enough.

I yanked his clothes off, he pulled my dress over my head and slipped on a Magnum (jealous?) and gave me one of those quick, kinda-rough bangings that I wish for every so often. It wasn't a juvenile "BANG BANG BANG" rabbit sex because dude is actually legit at fucking and I always come first. But it was definitely one of those "Let's not waste 20 precious minutes before you go to work. Might as well have an orgasm, right?" I think my bed moved a few feet.

He got dressed while I was doing multiplication tables in the bathroom trying to pee (it works!) and then I walked him to the door and took a Sunday nap. I mean, really – is anything more perfect than that? I highly recommend it. Call up your dude, entice him over and tell him Jillian said so.

13

27 Men Describe The Hottest Sext That Made Them Cum In Their Pants Immediately

Adrienne West

1. "My all time favorite sext said 'you're welcome any time, anywhere.' That's the one I always think about."

– Pat, 25

2. "I had a crush on a coworker but I never did a thing about it until she left. We both got tipsy at her going away happy hour and went home. I started texting her and things heated up quickly. Finally, she sent me a picture of her boobs. I wrote back that they looked amazing, to which she responded 'not as good as they'd look with your cum on them.' I Ubered to her place immediately and we had the hottest sex ever."

– Andy, 24

3. "I'm super visual so the best sexts I get from my wife are pictures. It works out for me because she's kind of an exhibitionist. She'll sneak off into the bathroom at work and send me something naughty to brighten up my afternoon."

- Rick, 30

4. "When I was on a business trip my girlfriend Snapchatted me a picture of her in bed. The caption said 'thanks for the orgasm.' The idea of her in bed touching herself and thinking about me drove me crazy. I couldn't wait to get home and make her cum again."

- Justin, 27

4. "The first time I slept with my wife when we started dating was a week night because I remember being at work a few hours later when she sent me a message that said 'I came so hard last night you almost made me pass out.' I was pretty nervous about how the night went because it was a new thing, but I felt like a fucking rockstar after that. And I was happy she wasn't playing games and making me guess how she felt about me. I set up another date immediately and things just got better from there."

- Brad, 33

5. "I dated an art student. Once she said 'Come over tonight. Bring a sharpie and write "I love you" all over my body.' It was strange... but very fun."

- Leo, 25

6. "A girl once asked me to come over but it was late and I had work the next day so I politely declined. Over Snapchat she sent me a video of her getting herself off. The caption said 'down for round 2?' Watching her face in the video along with the invitation to see it again drove me crazy. I went over after all and the live show was even better."

– Mike, 23

7. "A FWB once said 'I've always thought it would be really hot to try anal.' Yup."

– Sean, 22

8. "My ex-girlfriend LOVED to tease me. She would start in the morning and send me a pic of the bra she was wearing that day, or her panties. Sometimes in the afternoon I'd get her bare breasts in her company's bathroom. In-between she'd describe how she was going to suck on my balls and get very specific about all the places she wanted her tongue to be as soon as we saw each other. I kept getting hard at my work which was annoying, but god I miss her."

– Brian, 31

9. "I broke up with my ex-girlfriend but I couldn't stop fucking her for an entire year because she would text me things like 'I'm still thinking about the way your face looks when I'm swallowing your cum. I need to see it again.' How can you say no to that?"

– Danny, 25

10. "I had been having so much fun hooking up with this girl for the past few months. We were only 'dating' in the most casual sense of the word but we always had a great time together. One day she sent me a text that said 'I think I'm in

love with your cock.' It was so perfect, it turned me on while also making me laugh."

- Jason, 28

11. "She said 'tell me again why you're not cumming down my throat right now?' She had a good point."

- Adam, 29

12. "It was a picture of her and her best friend laying in bed and lifting up their shirts so I could see both of their boobs. It was supposed to be more silly than sexual, but holy shit this is my number one favorite memory. I still think about it all the time when I jerk off."

- David, 35

13. "I was a late bloomer so I was always insecure about how I was with women in my 20s. Then one girl sent me a text that said 'your dick is literally perfect and I would ride it every morning if I could.' Now whenever I feel insecure, I think about that text to psych myself up."

- Sam, 32

14. "She won't admit it but when she was intoxicated once my girlfriend told me she wanted to 'drink my cum for breakfast, lunch, and dinner.' She thinks it was too nasty or explicit or whatever but her enthusiasm for me is hot as fuck."

- Brandon, 25

15. "My high school girlfriend once sent 'you got it Daddy.'

She didn't mean it sexually at the time but… that's how I figured out that that's something that does it for me."

– Jake, 23

16. "Out of nowhere the girl I'm dating said 'I want you to fuck my face.' She's a preacher's daughter."– Josh, 26

17. "My cock is average size, it's nothing special. But a girl I was casually sleeping with got drunk and told me no one has "filled" her like I did. Instant boner, forever confidence."

– Rob, 28

18. "The day before we left for our first vacation together my then girlfriend sent me a picture of her ass in her new bikini and said "we better not come home until your handprint is on this ass." The girl loves to be spanked."

– Pete, 36

19. "I once date a conservative girl and for some reason I was the one that brought out her freak side. She would text me the nastiest shit like 'I can't decide what I need more right now, your cum in my mouth or your cum in my pussy' and 'I want you to teach me how to make you cum in under two minutes.' The fact that she was so eager and open and *freaky* really turned me on."

– John, 30

20. "On a first date with a girl I met at a bar I felt my phone buzz so I looked at my texts quickly. It was from her. It said

'I'm already wet'. I've never been so horny at a coffee shop before."

– Carl, 27

21. "We've been married five years and "come home so I can fuck your brains out" still works wonders for me."

– Steve, 33

22. "I saw the Packers lost. Blow job?"

– Ed, 29

23. "One night my girlfriend and I were sleeping at our own apartments. She Snapchatted me "I'm about to fuck myself so hard with my toy and think of you." We'd never done anything like it before, but we ended up sending each other pictures and masturbating to each other for hours. It was incredibly hot even though we were kind of used to having sex at that point."

– Justin, 33

24. "I had a terrible day at work and texted my FWB about it. She responded "I'll fuck you until you can't remember it if you come over later." Not only did I instantly forget about what a bad mood I was supposed to be in, but we had a lot of good sex later."

– Tom, 30

25. "I like it when a girl texts me that she's sore the next day. I feel like a champion stud and I know I made her feel good too."

– Nick, 27

26. "Out of nowhere one of my (I thought platonic) girl friends texted me "by the way I'm really good at sucking dick and I don't want to get out of practice, lmk if you could help a girl out." I totally admired her confidence. We started seeing each other occasionally just for sex and it was so hot to have this dirty secret none of our mutual friends knew about."

– Paul, 34

27. "She just said 'Cum over and don't say anything, I want to blow you for at least a half hour before I make you cum harder than you ever have before.' She delivered and it's my favorite memory."

– Matt, 31

Thought Catalog, it's a website.
www.thoughtcatalog.com

Social
facebook.com/thoughtcatalog
twitter.com/thoughtcatalog
tumblr.com/thoughtcatalog
instagram.com/thoughtcatalog

Corporate
www.thought.is

www.ingramcontent.com/pod-product-compliance
Lightning Source LLC
Chambersburg PA
CBHW050511290526
45786CB00007B/2519